I Have Chiari But It Doesn't Have Me

By Donna Mott
Illustrated by Karen Taylor

For Luke, who is my own super strong Chiari warrior
who taught me what living by faith day by day looks like.
And to Stephanie, another Chiari warrior who kept me from
crumbling that first day.

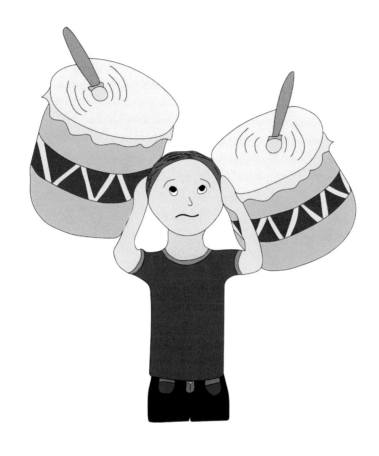

My head sometimes hurts like the pounding of a drum.

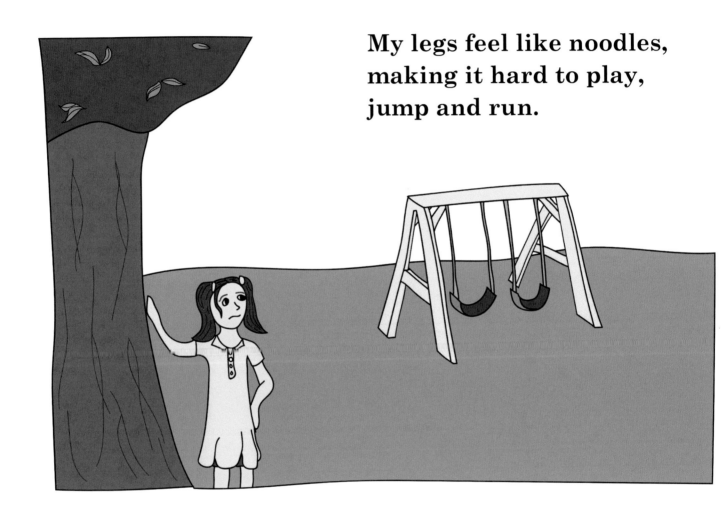

My legs feel like noodles, making it hard to play, jump and run.

I get the dizzies, see weird with my eyes.

Sometimes I just want to sleep, scream or cry!

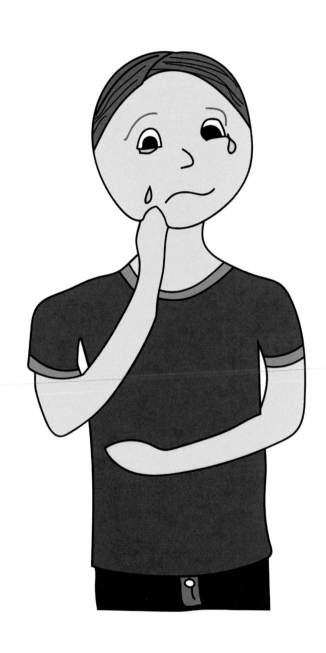

So, mom took me to a doctor for help to explain

why I feel so bad and guess what?

It's my brain!

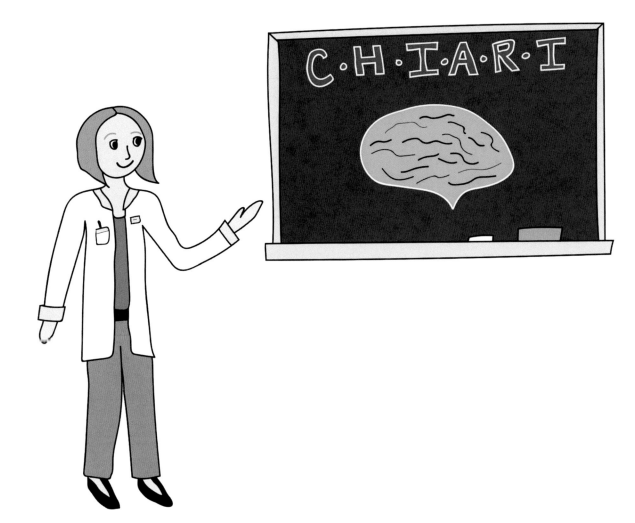

My brain is so smart.

My brain is so wise.

The doc says it's bigger than most my size.

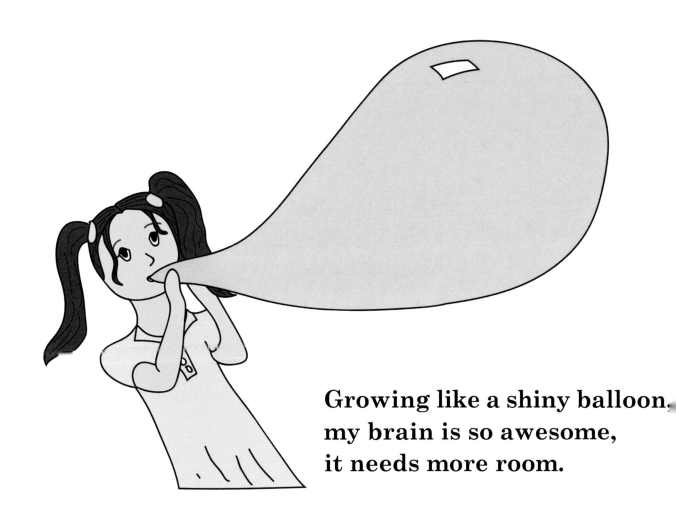

Growing like a shiny balloon,
my brain is so awesome,
it needs more room.

I'm running out of space in my head.

It's like a small room with a very big bed.

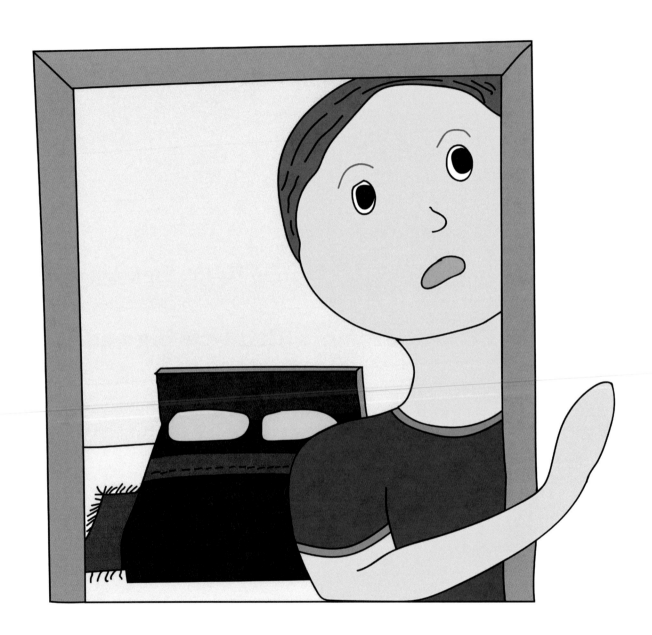

The name for it may sound a bit funny.

I think that it's called, what's the word?

Chiari.

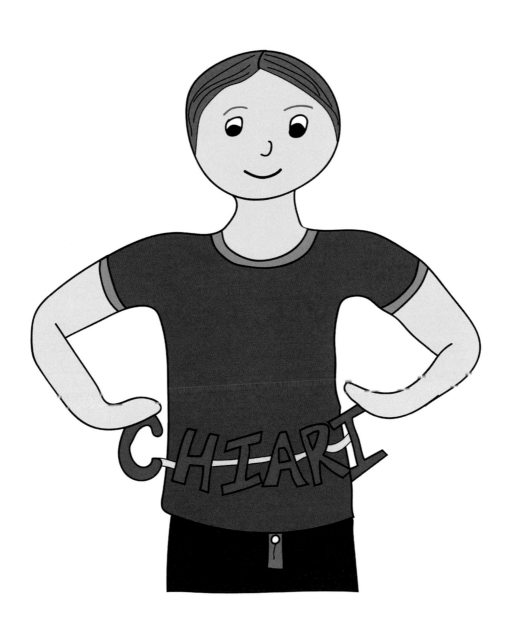

Let me show you again so you can plainly see
Look right here.

KEY-ARGHH-EE

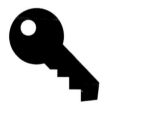  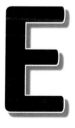

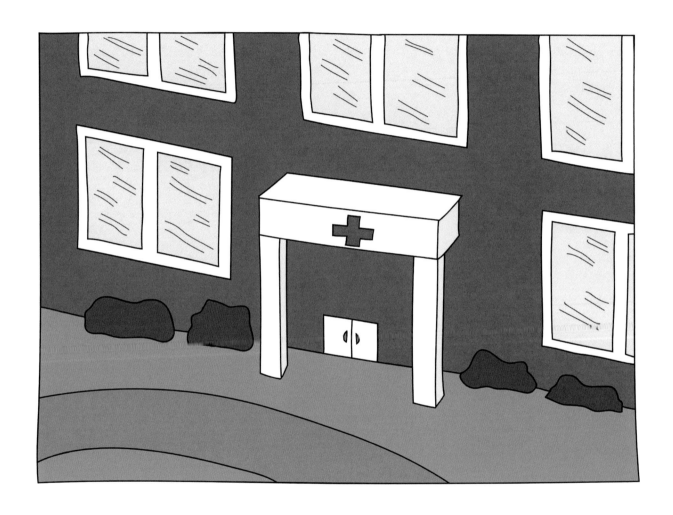

I might need a trip to the hospital for tests.

I might need surgery,
medicine and rest.

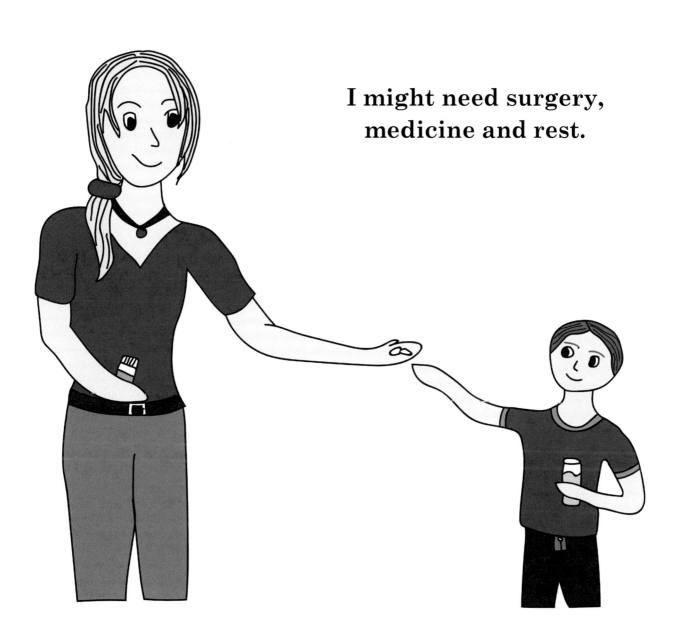

I am determined to do whatever

That I need to do to help me feel better.

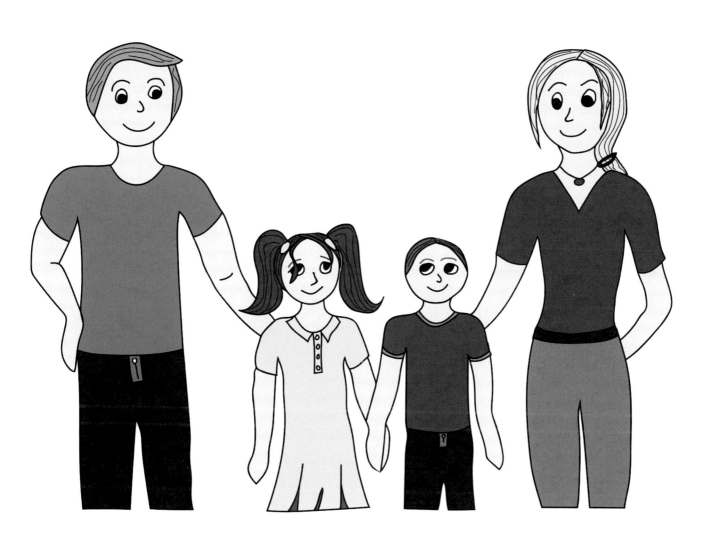

With my family and doctors to help me, I'm set.

I'm brave and I'm strong
and I'll beat this thing yet.

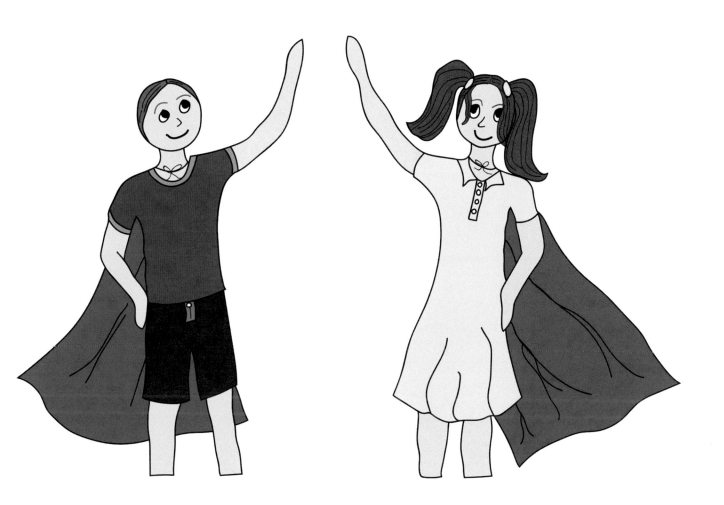

I'm a super hero, a warrior, you'll see.
I have Chiari,

but it doesn't have me!

Made in the USA
Middletown, DE
04 August 2021

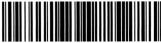

45343117R00015